The Adams Recovery Center Workbook

A COMPREHENSIVE GUIDE TO THE PROCESS OF HEALING ADDICTION

KiCam PROJECTS

Special thanks to Kimberly Kembel of Adams Recovery Center.

Cover and book design by Mark Sullivan

ISBN 978-0-9991581-8-0

Printed in the United States of America

Published by KiCam Projects
www.KiCamProjects.com

TABLE OF CONTENTS

INTRODUCTION | *v*

ABOUT ADAMS RECOVERY CENTER | *vii*

SECTION ONE: ACCEPT, REFLECT, COMMIT | *1*

CHAPTER ONE: *The Tipping Point* | *3*
CHAPTER TWO: *Choosing the Right Treatment* | *7*
CHAPTER THREE: *Trusting the Process* | *13*
CHAPTER FOUR: *Playing the Victim Role* | *17*
CHAPTER FIVE: *Wearing a Mask* | *21*
CHAPTER SIX: *People-Pleasing* | *23*
CHAPTER SEVEN: *Avoiding Dangerous Comparisons* | *27*
CHAPTER EIGHT: *Managing Your Anger* | *31*
CHAPTER NINE: *Forgiving Yourself and Others* | *35*
CHAPTER TEN: *Dealing with Death* | *39*
CHAPTER ELEVEN: *The Issue with Cross-Addiction* | *43*

SECTION TWO: ADDICTION, RECOVERY, CHANGE | *47*

CHAPTER ONE: *Setting Expectations after Treatment* | *49*
CHAPTER TWO: *Finding Sober Supports* | *53*
CHAPTER THREE: *Assessing Your Relationships* | *55*
CHAPTER FOUR: *Breaking Free of Codependence* | *59*
CHAPTER FIVE: *Battling Boredom* | *63*
CHAPTER SIX: *Encountering Temptation* | *67*
CHAPTER SEVEN: *Common Questions and Thinking Errors* | *71*

SECTION THREE: ASSESS, REBUILD, CONNECT | *75*

CHAPTER ONE: *A Quick Overview* | *77*
CHAPTER TWO: *Rebuilding Trust* | *79*
CHAPTER THREE: *Living with Integrity* | *83*
CHAPTER FOUR: *Navigating New Firsts* | *87*
CHAPTER FIVE: *Avoiding Becoming Overwhelmed* | *91*

Chapter Six: *Managing Family Dynamics* | *95*
Chapter Seven: *Handling the Holidays* | *99*
Chapter Eight: *Connecting to Your Passion* | *103*
Chapter Nine: *Medical Care and the Importance of Healthy Thinking* | *107*
Chapter Ten: *Aftercare Options* | *111*

RESOURCES | *115*

PAGES FOR JOURNALING | *117*

INTRODUCTION

We are delighted you have picked up this workbook!

Our hope is that no matter where or how you're using this material—in one of our treatment centers, in another treatment center, or on your own—you find this to be a meaningful guide as you navigate the challenges you'll face in getting and staying sober. Though this workbook won't "cure" anyone's addiction, we believe it is a powerful tool you can rely on day to day to overcome the obstacles most individuals face during treatment and in early sobriety.

If you're using this workbook on its own, great! We encourage you to take time with the reflection questions and really be honest with yourself in your answers. The deeper you dig, the more valuable the process will be, just as with anything in recovery.

We also recommend you make use of the three books that serve as source material for this workbook. Though the chapters are summarized here, you'll find greater detail—and possibly greater personal clarity—in the original texts, all of which are written in the same down-to-earth, easy-to-apply style you'll find in this workbook.

Whatever path you choose, we applaud you for taking these steps to better your life and the lives of your loved ones. Sobriety isn't easy, but it is *so* worth the work! We're honored that you've chosen Adams Recovery Center (ARC) to support you as you take what probably will be the most important journey of your life.

About Adams Recovery Center

ARC is an agency dedicated to change. We are a separate-gender drug and alcohol treatment program that offers residential, intensive outpatient, and individual counseling services, as well as a detoxification program. Our program is a modified Therapeutic Community running the Hazelden clinical curriculum. We use the latest evidence-based practices and incorporate cognitive behavioral therapy, rational-emotive behavior therapy, and behavior therapy to maximize client gains in the program. Our inpatient program is designed for an approximate one-hundred-eighty-day stay. Our staff includes drug and alcohol counselors and mental health counselors, as well as two medical doctors and a registered nurse.

ARC embraced the Therapeutic Community model due to its renowned success worldwide. The Therapeutic Community is recognized and endorsed by the United States federal government. Within the T.C., clients (called "sisters," "brothers," or "the family" collectively) come out of their denial and into acceptance regarding their substance abuse. Clients expose their thinking errors and learn how to look at people, places, and things differently. The T.C. is a residential hierarchy in which every resident has a job (for example, cleaning the kitchen, taking out the trash, inspecting the dorms, etc.). Clients engage in several hours of group therapy per day, in addition to individual counseling and case management.

We do not believe that one size fits all when it comes to treatment, and we do not believe we can simply hand clients answers. Instead, we help them find their own.

When a client has made sufficient evident clinical and personal progress at ARC, the client graduates and is referred for aftercare. We make sure our graduates feel comfortable and confident in themselves and in their aftercare plans.

Many of our clients go on to live successful lives free of substances, and we love hearing from these clients and celebrating their continued progress.

Our Staff

The staff at ARC comprises individuals who are certified or licensed in various disciplines. All clinical staff hold, at the minimum, certifications as chemical dependency counselors (CDCA) in the state of Ohio. Most staff are licensed as chemical dependency counselors (LCDC, Level 2 and Level 3), and others hold Licensed Independent Chemical Dependency Counselor (LICDC) designations.

Multiple staff members hold the LICDC-CS, which is the clinical supervisory endorsement—the highest form of chemical dependency licensure in Ohio.

We come from various counseling backgrounds, from a variety of schools of thought. We draw from cognitive behavioral therapy, behavior therapy, rational-emotive behavior therapy, reality therapy, choice therapy, existential/gestalt therapy, and other diverse therapeutic orientations, which allows multiple techniques and interventions to be used.

Several members of our staff contributed to this workbook and the related series of books in order to provide a broad spectrum of experience and approaches.

SECTION ONE

Accept, Reflect, Commit

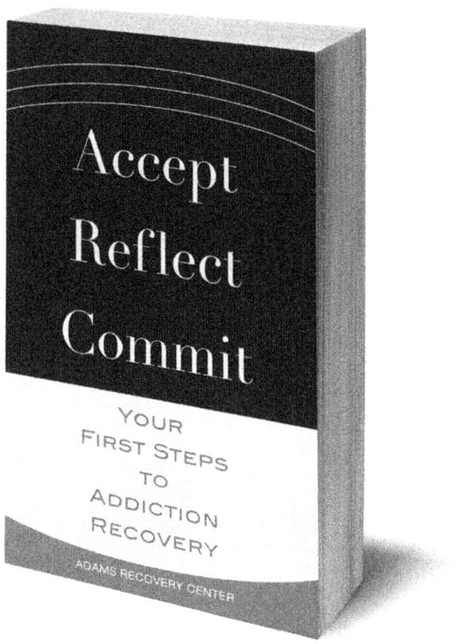

CHAPTER ONE

The Tipping Point

This chapter helps you determine whether your substance use is a problem. Addiction is defined as the state of being physically and mentally dependent on something. For some people, addiction slowly happens over time. They might have started using because it was "fun," but then their body and brain became dependent on the substance and they started to see the substance use as "normal."

Is there a problem? This appears to be a simple question, but for some it is hard to answer. One way to break it down is to ask yourself: "Is my substance use causing harm in my life or causing negative effects?" If the answer is yes, then you have more to research.

Professionals use the *Diagnostic and Statistical Manual of Mental Disorders (Fifth Edition)*, also known as the DSM5, to look at the criteria that could indicate a substance addiction. Some of the criteria relate to craving a drug, taking the drug in larger amounts over a longer period, spending a significant amount of time obtaining the drug or recovering from the drug, and experiencing withdrawal symptoms. For the complete list, see pages four and five of *Accept, Reflect, Commit*. The list has eleven specific criteria, and if you relate to at least two of them, then you could be diagnosed with a substance-use disorder. The DSM5 is just one piece of diagnosing a substance-use disorder; professionals also take other things into account, so it is important to *not* diagnose yourself. Instead, seek professional help.

The chapter also addresses interventions, which are fairly new. Thus, there is not a lot of information on them. Some things we do know are that interventions can bring families together, they are emotional, they do not always work, and they can be more effective with a professional leader. The main purpose of an intervention is for family or friends to express their concerns with the addicted person. In active addiction, you might not see how your addiction has affected others around you.

If you are a loved one trying to help someone in addiction, there is a way to communicate your concerns in a healthy manner. Try saying something along the lines of, "We have been late on paying our bills over the past several months because most of our money is going to drugs" instead of "Your addiction is causing money troubles." Make sure you are not placing blame and that you are coming from a place of care and concern. Interventions are just a starting point; the motivation to change comes from the follow-through by loved ones when the intervention is over.

Enabling is a problematic behavior that can prevent follow-through. Enabling is defined as giving someone the permission or ability to do something. For example, allowing an addicted person to continue his negative behavior with no consequences is enabling. If an addict is getting high in his mother's house and the mother says, "If you don't get help for your addiction, you will be kicked out," but then she does not follow through, the enabled addict believes such threats are empty. There are many other forms of

enabling, such as providing money, lending a car or other resource, or calling in "sick" for someone who is really high or hungover. Most loved ones do these things because they think they are being helpful and/or they do not want to lose the addict. But when you enable someone, you lose him to his drug of choice. Addiction can kill, and it will destroy everything over time.

QUESTIONS

1. After reviewing the criteria from the DSM5, do you think you have an issue with substance abuse? What criteria specifically relate to you? Reflect on a time when the criteria have applied to you. Example: Craving a drug—"I wake up every morning wanting to use, and I cannot do anything else until I get high."

2. When did you realize you were struggling with addiction?

3. If your family/friends had an intervention with you, how would it go? Who would be there? How would you respond? Would you follow through with getting help? Would you think it was a waste of time? If so, why?

4. How has your addiction affected your loved ones?

5. Who is enabling you, or are you the enabler? What can you do to stop this behavior?

CHAPTER TWO

Choosing the Right Treatment

When looking for a treatment program that works best for you, it is important to know what your options are. Not all treatments are the same, and not every treatment is going to benefit you. When starting your search for a treatment center, it is important to look at the philosophy of the center, the requirements, and the payment methods. Some treatment centers are paid for out of your own pocket, and you do not want to graduate treatment with a large amount of debt. Another thing to consider is that sometimes insurance companies cover only a certain amount of days, which could lead to you leaving treatment before your graduation day. If you do not have insurance, there are places like Job and Family Services that can help you.

Treatment programs are probably never going to be exactly what you want, but they can help you get what you need. It is important to go into treatment with realistic expectations. Treatment is not going to provide you all the answers; it is not a "cure." Treatment is going to be hard and challenging, and you will be expected to put in the work to get on the path to sobriety. No one is going to do the work for you.

Finding the right treatment can be frustrating. Use the information below to help you figure out the type of treatment you would be most likely to benefit from:

Detoxification: The main focus is to help individuals detox from substances. Going through withdrawal is difficult and is one of the reasons people walk out of treatment. Detoxing for alcohol and benzodiazepines can be deadly, so it is recommended to seek medical detox. Detox treatments are generally shorter, lasting anywhere from three to fourteen days. Generally, this is not enough time to fully recover, but it is a great first step.

Outpatient Treatment: This type of treatment can vary at different locations. The main focus is group and/or individual counseling. Our individualized program will require multiple groups a week, whereas some will require only one hour of individual counseling per week. Outpatient treatment is generally recommended for individuals who have been sober for at least three months and have the support to stay sober. Most people attend outpatient after they have completed residential.

Residential Treatment: In this case, an individual can live at a treatment center for a particular amount of time. Residential treatment can provide structure and a safe environment for individuals who are struggling to remain sober on their own. These treatment centers can be drastically different, so consider the list below when looking for residential programs:

- Structure
- Program type
- Counseling

- Interactions with others
- Facility
- Privileges

There are negative aspects to residential treatment. Some people cannot afford it, so it is important to check with your insurance company to see what is covered. Individuals in residential treatment also must figure out who will watch their children, pay their bills, watch over the house, etc.

Medication Assisted Treatment (MAT): This is the use of medication to help with withdrawal and/or cravings. Along with the medication, individuals are generally required to attend outpatient or residential treatment to help look at deeper issues related to the substance use. MAT is comforting when entering treatment because withdrawal is a scary part of getting sober. But MAT can be viewed as a setback. Some individuals and/or their families see it as substituting one drug for another, and it is possible to become dependent. It is important to process your thoughts and feelings with your medical provider. Below is the type of medication that can be offered for opiate and/or alcohol addiction:

- Buprenorphine is a low-dose opioid that assists with cravings and minimizes withdrawal symptoms. This comes in a pill form or a film strip that helps blocks the effect of an opiate, which discourages people from wanting to use. This medication has a low chance of addiction and can be prescribed and then taken at home. Just because there is a low chance of addiction does not mean that it cannot happen. If buprenorphine is abused and the medication is no longer available, it can cause withdrawal symptoms.
- Methadone is similar to buprenorphine. It is an opioid that helps with cravings and withdrawal. It can be given in a pill form or as an oral concentrate (liquid form). This does not have the same blocker effect that buprenorphine has, and it can be highly addictive. This medication is dispensed at a facility, and individuals need to visit the facility daily to get the proper dose. Stopping methadone can cause withdrawal symptoms.
- Naltrexone completely blocks the effects of opiates and can discourage someone from using again. This medication can be taken in pill form or as a monthly injection. Naltrexone does not give a euphoric feeling, so it isn't likely to be abused. This medication does not completely block the effects of alcohol, but it does interrupt the pleasurable feeling individuals get from drinking. There are minimal side effects from Naltrexone.

Sober Support Groups: It is important to understand that support groups are not a type of treatment; they are simply there for support. They provide a helping hand for people who are struggling with addiction. These groups consist of Alcoholics Anonymous, Narcotics Anonymous, Celebrate Recovery, SMART Recovery, Secular Sobriety, etc. Meetings take place daily or weekly and in different locations. These meetings have different philosophies and cover different topics. Support meetings also have sober social events to help people in recovery build more of a sober network.

Sober Living: This is also not a type of treatment, but sober living arrangements are helpful. Many people seek sober living to help meet the need for structure. Sober living houses can have individuals who

are new to sobriety, as well as individuals who have been sober for months or years. Different sober houses have different rules and regulations. For some, you might have to attend an outpatient program or go to a certain number of meetings a week. Looking into the rules and regulations of each program is important. Some people need more structure than others, and some sober living might not have any rules. The latter could provide an unsafe environment that could lead to relapse. Sober living can help transition into that "normal lifestyle."

Most people end up choosing more than one type of treatment. People might enter residential, then graduate, go to sober living, and attend an outpatient program. There is no evidence that one treatment is better than another. To find the right treatment option for you, it is important to get an assessment completed. In an assessment, a professional will ask multiple questions about your life and drug use in order to recommend the appropriate level of care.

QUESTIONS

1. What are your thoughts and feelings toward treatment? Are you scared? Are you frustrated? Do you think you can do this alone? Is treatment a waste of time?

2. What do you want to gain from a treatment program? What are your goals and expectations?

3. If you were to decide to do MAT, which medication would you want prescribed? Why?

4. Make a pro vs. con list on each type of treatment that was discussed: detoxification, outpatient, residential, MAT, support groups, and sober living.

PROS	CONS

5. What is your ideal treatment combination? If this does not work, what is another combination you could try?

CHAPTER THREE

Trusting the Process

Chapters two and three go hand in hand, because as you consider treatment, you want to choose a program you truly believe in. That will make it easier for you to trust the process. To "trust the process" means to allow things to work out how they should. This concept can be simple but also complicated. It comes down to control.

Think about your active addiction. You took time to control the chaotic lifestyle you were living; you might have manipulated, hustled, or stolen to get your drug of choice. That gave you a sense of control. When you enter treatment, you are required to follow the program's rules, regulations, and policies. This can bring up difficult questions that give you the sense you are losing control. That puts you of out your comfort zone. When you are out of your comfort zone, your feelings might cause you to think things such as "I don't need to listen to these people" or "I should go back to when things were easy." Giving in to these thoughts can cause you to leave treatment before change has begun. When you give up control, you'll find that sobriety can be more easily achieved because you are willing to take difficult steps to start a new life.

A common misconception about the phrase "trust the process" is believing you can sit back, relax, and wait for things to change. Finding balance with control is key. You need to reflect on what is in your control versus what is out of your control and then put it all together to create a new life. This will help you face challenges head on, which is part of life for everyone.

When challenging situations occur in treatment, it might make you doubt the program. Before reacting based on that doubt, ask yourself these questions:

- What role is control trying to play in this situation?
- In what ways could this be a valuable experience?
- How can I learn and grow from this experience?
- How can I apply this to my life outside of treatment?
- In the long run, will this matter?

If you consider these questions, you are challenging your perspective and allowing yourself to experience difficult or negative emotions. Allowing yourself to do this enables you to stop, reflect, and continue to trust the process. When you change your perspective, you get to see the bigger picture and not be focused on a minor detail. Trusting the process is having faith during difficult times, which will allow you to continue to move forward.

QUESTIONS

1. What scares you about "trusting the process"?

2. Now that you have an idea of what treatment you would like to try, what does your treatment process look like?

3. What did you control in your active addiction, and what are you trying to control now?

4. Reflect on a life situation you are experiencing right now. What is in your control? What is out of your control?

5. What are you willing to do—physically, mentally, and emotionally—to achieve sobriety?

CHAPTER FOUR

Playing the Victim Role

Life is awful. I am all alone and no one cares. I am a terrible person and my life will never get better.

If these thoughts sound familiar to you, then you're familiar with the victim mentality. The victim role is a way of thinking that makes you feel awful, and that type of mind-set makes it hard to become sober. You start to believe the world is against you, and you want the world to feel bad for you. If you choose to stay a victim, you're basically giving yourself permission to use drugs and/or alcohol.

Being a victim does have some benefits, but they are short term. Victim mentality is connected with manipulation. When you manipulate someone, you are getting that person to do what you want. Essentially, you are getting that person to enable your unhealthy behavior, which traps you in a vicious cycle of never-ending use and abuse.

Victim mentality is displayed in various ways. For example, it can be connected to low self-esteem, which makes it difficult to pursue goals and follow through on things. Victim behavior also can be displayed by those who appear to be "a good person in a bad world." Such individuals consider themselves caretakers, and they will do anything when it comes to helping others—but they do it for personal gain. If they don't get the attention, respect, or whatever other outcome they seek, then they become resentful and decry the world as unfair. Again, the underlying issue is the desire for control.

Some clients feel like victims because they truly have suffered through a traumatic experience, such as childhood abuse, domestic violence, sexual assault, war, etc. If you have experienced trauma, then you could be holding on to it because you feel like it defines who you are. That hinders your ability to move forward. It is not easy to get over these experiences, but when you hold on to them, you are allowing yourself to be a victim. With traumatic experiences, using drugs and alcohol can block the painful emotions and/or memories, allowing you to feel "normal." Of course, that normality is only superficial.

One way to combat the victim mind-set is through reframing, which is challenging your perceptions and thought patterns to become open-minded about viewing something differently. You might call it walking in someone else's shoes. As we grow up, we develop our own way of seeing the world, which not everyone else shares. The chapter uses a window as an example. The victim mentality is like having bars over the window, which partially block your view. When you look at the world through other people's windows, you get a different perspective. You also can shatter your window and create a new one based off new personal views you choose to add into your life.

Another way to overcome the victim mentality is to practice gratitude—being thankful for the things you have. Making a gratitude list daily can help you become humble, whereas the victim mentality makes you believe that everything in life is terrible. You feel grateful when you focus more on the positive than

on the negative. Gratitude is also related to empowerment. When you feel empowered, you regain your sense of control. Empowerment enables you to learn more about the talents, abilities, and interests you have been pushing to the side over the years.

QUESTIONS

1. Describe a time when you displayed a victim mentality. What are some phrases you used?

2. What traumas have you experienced? Are you allowing those experiences to have power over you?

3. How can you practice reframing? To whom can you go for a different perspective?

4. Make a gratitude list. (Examples: I am grateful for food, a roof over my head, clothes, running water, etc.)

5. What are some of your talents, abilities, and/or interests?

CHAPTER FIVE

Wearing a Mask

If someone asked you who you are, what would be your response? You might just say your name, but that is not what we mean. This question is really asking you to look at yourself down to the core and take time to figure out your identity.

In active addiction, you slowly started to lose your identity. Think about the things you wouldn't have done or said if you'd been sober. In the beginning of your addiction, you might have pretended to blend in to appear "cool," but then over time the pretending became a way of living. That is not who you truly are. But when the masks are removed, you could notice feelings of frustration and confusion over figuring out who you are. That's part of what a good treatment program will help you work through.

You might be wondering what the difference is when it comes to wearing a mask versus playing a role. The main difference is genuineness or authenticity. In your life, you might play the role of sibling, parent, spouse, friend, or child. In each role, you have different requirements, so you adjust your behavior accordingly. For example, you might speak differently to your grandparents than you do to your friends. It doesn't mean you aren't being the real you; you're just tailoring how you act to be appropriate for a given situation.

When you wear a mask, however, you are not being true to yourself. Lying, for instance, is a form of mask-wearing. Manipulation is another. You might wear masks because you are trying to gain something for your own benefit and get another person to perceive you differently. You might be using the mask to hide (or to hide *from*) your true identity because it is more comfortable than having others see the real you. Over time, wearing a mask stops you from moving forward. By letting go of the mask, you can trust the process and allow your true identity to come to the surface.

The first step in breaking free of the mask is figuring out which mask or masks you're wearing. One way to do that is by writing an autobiography, beginning from the day you were born and continuing through today. Once you've written it, you can reflect on your life and see when your behavior started to change and when you started wearing masks. The autobiography is just a starting point; learning about yourself is a lifelong process.

The bottom line is to trust the process and break free from the lies you have been trying to hold together to please others. Embrace this opportunity to become who you really are.

QUESTIONS

1. Who were you in active addiction? Did you use slang words or wear a certain type of clothing? How are these things different now that you are sober?

2. Use some of the blank pages in the back of this workbook to write your autobiography. There is no right or wrong way to do this. This assignment is about *your* life. Start with your name and where you are from and go from there. Now that you have written your autobiography, go back and look at where your life started to change. Assess your behaviors. What types of masks did/do you wear, and what does each mask do for you? Write your answers below.

CHAPTER SIX

People-Pleasing

It's nice to lend a helping hand to someone in need, but at what point does helping others become dangerous? This concept is called people-pleasing, a type of behavior that can be dangerous and possibly hinder you from moving forward in your sobriety. A basic thing to understand about people-pleasing is that it is not always black and white. This is connected to the way you think. Have you ever heard yourself or others say things like "always" and "never"? That type of thinking places you in an unrealistic box, which makes it hard to stay motivated. Think back to the window example in chapter four. If you are viewing everything as black and white, you are not allowing yourself to consider other perceptions. You need to embrace the gray area.

Most people say they help others because it is the right thing to do, but we challenge you to examine your motives. After reflecting, you might see you are helping others only to gain something for a benefit: "I'll scratch your back if you scratch mine." That's simply manipulation, often accompanied by sneaky behavior. Think about it: No one is going to come out and say, "I will do this for you, but I am only doing it so I can rub it in your face months from now." It's more likely that you'll hear something along the lines of: "Remember when I helped you out three months ago and I really put myself on the line? Now you aren't going to help me? I can't believe you would do this—shows you what type of person you are! … Oh, now you'll do it? Great!" This example is manipulation at its finest. The bottom line is to check your intentions before doing something to help others.

People-pleasing is also connected to street-like behavior. When you are on the streets, you sometimes might not have money, so you trade for other things. For example, you might let a drug dealer stay with you in return for free drugs. This can be dangerous because your house could be turned into a trap house. You're then stuck in a bad situation. A similar phenomenon occurs in treatment sometimes, when you let someone's bad behavior slide in exchange for that person doing the same for you. That keeps you *and* the other person stuck. You might get what you want in the moment, but ultimately, it's an unhealthy situation.

People-pleasing and street-like behavior also relate to "snitching." In addiction, you learn that "snitching" can get you hurt—or worse. So, you turn a blind eye to others' illegal, unhealthy activity by justifying, minimizing, and rationalizing. You've learned to believe that telling the truth is against the code. But in recovery, you have an opportunity to change your mentality and your environment, to be around people who are going to support you, not harm you, when you do the right thing.

When you encourage others to hold you accountable, you are protecting your sobriety. When you take the steps to have a safer environment, you will no longer tolerate harmful behaviors and negative thinking patterns. Doing this, you might make people around you unhappy, but you will be able to focus

on your own happiness and your own goals. To get out of the people-pleasing habit, you have to make sure you have enough time for *you* before giving your time to others. It is okay to say no. For example, if someone asks you for a ride but you have only enough gas to get to work later, then you need to say no. If you gave this person a ride, you probably would not make it to work and then would suffer the consequences. You cannot take care of others if you cannot take care of yourself. If you are not 100 percent, you cannot give 100 percent.

It is okay to be selfish in order to get well! Take this time to get your environment and mind-set together. Set boundaries, embrace the word "no," and check your behaviors. Ask yourself, are you doing a specific thing to help someone? To gain acceptance? To manipulate? Or is it a mixture? Taking a few moments to analyze your behaviors can help you kick your people-pleasing to the curb. People-pleasing is not a behavior that will keep you sober.

QUESTIONS

1. Describe a time when you demonstrated people-pleasing or when someone was trying to please you.

2. Break down your response from number one and figure out what form of people-pleasing you were experiencing (manipulation, street-like behavior, snitch mentality, or being overly helpful).

3. What are some examples of black-and-white thinking from your past?

4. What do you think about "snitching"? If you have a negative mind-set, is this something you are willing to change?

5. How can you work on providing a safe environment for yourself?

CHAPTER SEVEN

Avoiding Dangerous Comparisons

It is natural to compare yourself to others—you've been doing it since you were a kid! But when you compare yourself to others, you can start to create unrealistic expectations, which can become dangerous—especially in sobriety.

In early sobriety, you are in search of who you are without drugs, and you are seeking others who can help guide you in figuring things out. If you do not pay close attention to how you are seeking guidance, you could end up just molding yourself to be like another person. That's not helpful or healthful.

One thing most people do in early sobriety is compare their treatment to someone else's process. This is connected to black-and-white thinking and instant gratification. You might be comparing yourself because you have low self-esteem or because you want to be "cured" right away. This behavior can keep you from progressing. Treatments are individualized and move at their own pace, which can be hard to accept. It also might not feel "fair" to you, but nothing in life is fair, and sobriety is no exception. For example, maybe you've been in residential treatment for sixty days and have not gotten a day pass yet, but someone who's been in for only forty days has received a pass. Seems unfair, right? But consider, you might not truly understand what that other person is going through. Perhaps he received a day pass because a close family member has passed away. It's also possible for one person to make more progress in a shorter time than someone else does. Keeping yourself focused on *yourself* is hard, but necessary.

Other clients' progress has nothing to do with you, even if you and someone else are facing similar problems or have similar backgrounds. For instance, perhaps you and another client both were abused as a child. You could be struggling to accept your past while the other client has worked hard on finding acceptance and is moving forward. It's natural and common for people to be in different places. You simply have to keep putting in the work to reach your goals.

One of the biggest comparison culprits is social media. Everyone's life looks better in pictures, but not everything is as great as it seems. You might jump on Facebook and see a married couple away on a beach vacation. You think to yourself, "Oh, that looks so nice! I wish I were married and on the beach right now. Wow, they are lucky." But in reality, you know nothing about their daily struggles, conflicts, issues, or worries. Social media keeps us updated on our friends and family, but rarely does anyone put the complete truth out there for everyone to see. Many people use social media to make everything seem great and positive. In turn, that can cause you to focus on all the things you want and don't have. That leads you to play the victim role and brings on negative emotions such as guilt, shame, depression, etc. When these emotions come on suddenly and quickly, you could resort to using again if you do not have proper coping skills. Another way social media can lead to using is in the depiction of people you know

drinking or getting high. You can forget all the negatives about substance use and be tempted to go back to your old friends and your old behaviors.

You can use social media safely and still achieve your goals related to sobriety. Here are some tips:

- Delete unhealthy friends from your list.
- Recognize reality and remember that not everything you see is the truth.
- Limit your time on social media.
- Create a positive feed that inspires you. Join recovery groups or groups that post supportive quotes.
- Live in the moment.

Keep in mind, it's great to have a role model or sponsor to help you get sober and stay sober. But ultimately, you want to be you. Don't try to be just like someone else. *You* are enough, and your life is worth living.

QUESTIONS

1. Reflect on your childhood and teenage years. How did you compare yourself back then?

____

____

____

____

____

2. Recall a time in your sobriety that you have compared yourself to someone else. Why did you pick this person? What characteristics did this person exhibit that you liked or admired?

____

____

____

____

____

3. When you use social media, what do you think about? Are you comparing yourself? What emotions do you feel?

4. Plan your new social media usage.

    - Whom are you going to delete?

    - How can you cope when your mind starts to wander away from reality?

    - What is your time limit?

- What groups can you join to help keep a positive flow on your news feed?

____

____

- How can you reconnect with your new life without social media?

____

____

CHAPTER EIGHT

Managing Your Anger

Anger is a misunderstood emotion. It can be seen as negative because of the way people often express it. But the fact is, anger is natural—it's not something that needs to be "fixed." What can be changed is the way a person responds to the feeling of anger

Anger is like any other emotion: It is healthy to experience, and it exists on a spectrum at different times for different individuals. Anger can range from mild frustration to intense rage. As with other emotions, most people experience anger at least once a day, and that is healthy. Anger helps us learn about ourselves. It keeps our morals, values, and boundaries in line and helps us identify our thought patterns. Anger is actually a secondary emotion, meaning it's tied to or caused by other underlying feelings. Here is the example from the book: "A past client became furious when her father asked what she planned to do post-treatment. After processing, the client discovered that her anger came along with shame and confusion because she did not know her plan yet. She felt fear, too; she was afraid of life after treatment." In this example, fear, shame, and confusion are the primary emotions that caused the client to feel and express anger. Situations like this one show why understanding your emotions is so important when new to sobriety. If you are still trying to numb your emotions, you are not really living and experiencing your life. This concept is connected to bottling feelings. Pretending that emotions do not exist or that something did not happen is only keeping yourself stuck. When you remain stuck, you don't develop healthy coping skills to move forward with your life. Thus, when a challenge comes your way, you're likely to resort to using to cope with the issue.

People often mix up anger and aggression, but there's a big difference: Anger is a feeling; aggression is a behavior. It is okay to feel anger, but aggression can become violent and cause problems. Acting aggressively is a learned behavior and can be changed, even when you're angry. Reflect on your upbringing. How were you raised when it comes to anger and aggression? Were you taught to talk sternly but calmly when dealing with an issue? Were you taught to fight it out to prove you were right? Or were you taught to just walk away and not say anything? Whatever the case, you can always learn to change your behavior.

When it comes to anger, you can learn healthier ways to work through it. Research has shown that hitting a pillow, smashing something, or beating a punching bag only reinforces aggressive behavior. Those actions might prevent you from being aggressive toward another person, but they don't actually help you process or manage your anger. To develop true coping skills, start by looking closely at your anger. Ask yourself:

1. What makes you angry? Take a daily inventory of times when you feel anger. The purpose of this is to help you figure out your own patterns.

2. What are your cues? Pay attention to these four areas:
   - Physical: heavy breathing, increased heart rate, face becoming red, etc.
   - Behavioral: clenching your fists, raising your voice, snarling, etc.
   - Emotional: Are you feeling sadness, frustration, disappointment, etc.?
   - Cognitive: Reflect on your thoughts. Are they aggressive? Are they negative self-talk?
3. What works for you? This is going to involve trial and error. Different coping skills are going to work for different situations. Start by trying these: deep breathing, soothing self-talk, and other forms of self-care. This is just a place to start. Anything healthy can become a coping skill.

In addition to developing coping skills, it is important to understand the different types of communication styles: passive, aggressive, passive-aggressive, and assertive. The example from the book is:

You are at the grocery store and the cashier rings up your order incorrectly. As he hands you your receipt, you notice the mistake. Your response is:

- Passive: You avoid any type of conflict. You might say something along the lines of, "Oh that's... um...okay...thank you."
- Aggressive: Your actions are loud, forceful, and accusatory. You will be direct with your feelings while belittling other people. You might say something such as, "Are you kidding me? This is wrong. It is off by $15. Are you stupid?"
- Passive-aggressive: This form is connected to sarcasm. You will try to avoid conflict but also get the last word in. You might say something such as, "Huh...I mean, sure, I guess I can pay a whole $15 more. Like, I am just rolling in cash right now, buddy."
- Assertive: This is the calm approach to solving a problem. You will be direct and comfortable with sharing your feelings. You also will listen to the other person. You might say, "Excuse me. There actually was another price displayed. It appears to be more on my receipt. Do you think you could take a look at this for me and change it? I would appreciate it."

Looking at these forms of communication, which one do you align with the most? If your communication is not assertive, what can you do to make adjustments? Being clear about your thoughts and emotions will lessen the chances of aggressive or argumentative behavior. It is challenging to be assertive all the time because of our emotional decision-making. But the more you practice assertive communication, the better you will get at it. Assertiveness will not just happen overnight. Like everything else, it is going to require trial and error.

Remember that anger is something you will come across just about every day and that it is healthy as long as it is expressed in a productive manner. Embracing and understanding your anger can help you achieve a calmer state of mind.

QUESTIONS

1. How do you express anger? What are the primary emotions that lead you to feel anger?

2. How were you raised to deal with anger or aggression?

3. Describe a time you felt anger and a time you displayed aggression. What was the difference?

4. Break down your anger:
   - What makes you angry?
   - What are your cues?
   - What works for you to manage your anger?

5. What is your communication style? When have you displayed passive, aggressive, passive-aggressive, and assertive styles? Describe the situations and recall what you said and how you said it. In situations when you were not assertive, what could you have done differently to communicate more effectively?

CHAPTER NINE

Forgiving Yourself and Others

When entering sobriety or treatment, you are going to be overwhelmed with emotions as you start to remember the things you did to others while in active addiction. One of the most common things clients want to work on is mending relationships with family and friends. The feelings that come with trying to fix a relationship could include guilt, shame, anger, etc. You also might feel like your family and friends are never going to trust or forgive you for your past. This chapter will not give you the steps for forgiveness, but it will challenge your ideas about forgiveness and present some thinking points.

Forgiveness is complicated, but it is doable. When seeking forgiveness, it is important to understand that it is going to look different with every situation and it is going to have challenges. There are going to be ups and downs, twist and turns. You are a human who has thoughts and emotions, and the people from whom you are seeking forgiveness also have thoughts and feelings. A lot of individuals who enter treatment think that because they are sober means their friends and family are just going to forgive them. Having the mind-set that forgiveness is that straightforward will only set you up for failure.

Forgiveness has its own timeline. Sometimes it happens quickly, and sometimes it takes longer than you would like. In addiction, you're used to instant gratification. In recovery, when things do not happen on your timeframe, you might feel as if you are running in circles and you might want to give up. Patience is a big part of the forgiveness process.

Just because you are forgiven does not mean that people forget. The concept of "forgive and forget" is actually dangerous. You cannot simply forget things—it doesn't work that way. When you want to forget about an event, you are also trying to forget the lesson that could have been learned from it. What you have experienced in life is what contributes to your behaviors and memories, which then connects to how you perceive things. If you get hurt or hurt someone else, you should take that experience to adjust your behaviors in order to prevent the same hurt from occurring again. The idea of "forgive and forget" also can give you the idea that it is okay to sweep things under the rug, but that allows you to continue displaying a negative behavior. A new way to look at forgiveness would be to "forgive and accept." When seeking forgiveness, we all would like for everything to go back to normal, but the reality is that things have changed. Hopefully, when things change, they change for the better; the relationship should become stronger, or it will eventually end. In order to forgive someone or for someone to forgive you, you must learn acceptance. When coming into acceptance, you are admitting what your reality is.

No one is going to go through this process for you. Following through with forgiveness is a choice, and it takes time both to get, and to give, forgiveness.

QUESTIONS

1. What is your definition of forgiveness?

2. From whom do you need to ask forgiveness? What was the situation? Why do you want/need forgiveness?

3. Is someone trying to get your forgiveness? What is stopping you from mending that relationship?

4. Have you recently been forgiven, or have you forgiven someone else? If so, how has your relationship changed? Is it better or worse?

5. How do you relate forgiveness to your addiction? Why is forgiveness important to you?

CHAPTER TEN

Dealing with Death

When entering sobriety, you will feel a flood of new emotions. In the process, you are going to start thinking of things that you did in your past that you are not proud of. You also might dwell on family or friends who are no longer alive. Dealing with death takes time to work through. Death is a part of life, and it is not going to go away just because you are working on sobriety. The good news: Looking at death from a different viewpoint can help you deal with it in real time.

Guilt, shame, and self-defeat are common reactions to losing someone. That can be because you used to use with the person, you were under the influence when the person died, or you missed the person's final days because you continued to use. When reflecting on these moments, you could start to create an unhealthy thought pattern. For example:

I should have been around more, and now he's gone. This statement is connected to regret. You might wish you had called more or spent more quality time with someone. During the time you did spend with this person, you were probably high or drunk. That can be hard to accept when you're new to sobriety. You cannot change your past, but you can change things in the future. So, in sobriety, spend more time with the ones you love and think about how you can do things differently than you used to.

She died of an overdose, and I was the one who introduced her to drugs. If this quote sounds familiar to you, then you are probably feeling responsible for someone's death. Thoughts that are connected to this could be: *Why did she have to die? Why wasn't it me? Do I deserve treatment right now?* These thoughts are important, and you do not want to ignore the influence you have on others, but look at reality: It is true that our actions and behaviors affect others, but humans make their own decisions. You might have introduced drugs to someone, but that person had the ability to choose whether or not to use drugs or alcohol. When you start to see the difference between influence and choice, it will lessen your guilt.

I was so messed up at the funeral, I don't even remember it. Or, *I was so messed up, I didn't even make it to the funeral.* Funerals are viewed differently by everyone. A lot of people see funerals as a chance to get "closure." The truth is, funerals are not magic, and most of the time they do not bring closure. Pain and loss don't go away just because you attend a funeral. Closure happens over time, and it can occur even if the person you are grieving is no longer living. By working on forgiveness (of both yourself and others) and pursuing your sobriety, you can honor your friend or loved one.

It's common to wonder how you're going to get through all of this. The easy way would be to use again and numb your feelings—but that's not an option. On the contrary, to deal with death, you can't ignore your emotions. That said, you don't want to obsess, either. Everyone handles death differently, so it can be helpful to understand the five stages of grief:

1. Denial and isolation: Not wanting to admit someone has passed is a part of this stage. Masking and bottling emotions also can occur at this stage.
2. Anger: The overwhelming feeling of the death can cause anger and blame.
3. Bargaining: Here, you try to regain control. For example, you might find yourself saying, "If I do *this*, maybe *that* won't happen."
4. Depression: This can be connected to sadness, regret, and shame.
5. Acceptance: You start to feel calm or a sense of peace. This does *not* mean you are happy the person is gone.

It is important to understand that these stages are not on a timeframe and that they can come and go in different orders.

One way to handle the loss of a loved one is through reconstruction, or changing your own perception. Take a look at a traumatic event from your past. Instead of thinking of it as traumatic, think about how strong you were in the moment to get through it.

Loss is something that affects our lives; it can make us or break us. You have the power and control to deal with death in a healthful manner. It is important to surround yourself with loved ones to help you feel strong in a time of sorrow.

QUESTIONS

1. When you think about a loved one who has passed away, what emotions do you feel?

2. What thought patterns have you experienced related to that death? What specific thoughts have you had? For example: *It should have been me that died and not him. I was the one who introduced him to drugs. He had kids, and I do not.*

3. How do you relate to the five stages of grief? What stage are you in? Why do you think you are in this stage? Are you ready to move to a different stage? (Remember, the stages are not on a timeframe and can go in any order.)

4. If you look at the death of someone close to you, how can you create a different perspective? Can you reconstruct the situation to find a positive angle?

5. Who are some healthy people you can surround yourself with if you're struggling with the death of a loved one?

CHAPTER ELEVEN

The Issue with Cross-Addiction

When it comes to cross-addiction, most people believe that if you are addicted to one thing, then you will become addicted to something else. This is not completely true. With more knowledge, you will be able to enjoy many activities in your future and not be afraid that you will get addicted to something.

Cross-addiction is real, but with the help of research, we all can understand it better. Columbia Medical University surveyed 34,000 people with a substance disorder and over the years found that people who ceased their first addiction were less likely to turn to another substance. That is because these people were able to work through their problems, establish healthy coping skills, and build a sober network. The others in the survey who developed another addiction never really stopped using their first substance.

In early recovery, you might feel the need to replace certain feelings or behaviors instead of learning healthy coping skills. The thing most people say is, "At least I am not using." This is true on some level, but other activities can be just as dangerous and could lead you back to using if not monitored correctly. Other activities can stimulate your brain just like drugs do. Let's take a look.

Alcohol: If you have abused drugs, then you might think to yourself, "I can still have a drink if I want and not get addicted." But this is not true for everyone. Ask yourself, why do you feel like you need to drink? What would you gain from drinking an alcoholic beverage? There is nothing saying you can never have a drink. Some people can have a drink and be just fine, while others feel like drinking will lead them back down the path to their addiction. At the end of the day, it is about personal awareness and making that decision for yourself.

Food: Eating is something we need to do to survive, but it also is a behavior that can trigger the brain's pleasure center. Research has shown that sugar is an addictive substance with tolerance and withdrawal symptoms. Think about a time when you were emotional and you "ate your feelings." This is a problem for a lot of people. If you excessively eat as a habit, you can develop health problems. A way to monitor this is to eat a healthy diet and treat yourself when it is deserved.

Sex and Pornography: Sex is an activity that stimulates the brain's pleasure center but can create a problem if done in excess. Figuring out a healthy sex life when new to sobriety can be challenging. Most people find sober sex to be scary after they've been used to having sex under the influence. Sober sex means feeling emotions and forming connections. Sex also has been known to be a coping mechanism or a way to continue addictive behaviors. The process of having sex is similar to the process of getting high or drunk: You have the desire, you search for a specific person, and you follow a sort of ritual that eventually leads to a positive feeling. Pornography also can be problematic in sobriety. It can cause major issues with personal relationships and also brings on unrealistic images of sex and sexuality. If you're struggling

with sex and pornography in sobriety, just know that it is normal and that others have experienced similar situations. There are ways to get help, such as post-treatment specific to sex and relationship issues.

Video Games and Technology: When it comes to video games, people tend to enjoy playing them because it helps them escape from reality. But when you play video games, you can get emotionally attached to certain characters online, which then can cause a detachment from real-life relationships. Video games can be dangerous if not used in moderation. Staying up late every night using energy drinks and playing video games is not moderation! Video games aren't the only potentially dangerous form of technology you'll encounter. Social media can be addictive and can take you away from the life going on around you. Make it a point to put your phone down and enjoy what's going on in the moment.

Money, Shopping, and Gambling: You might experience an overwhelming feeling when it comes to money. This feeling can be connected with how your money was used in your active addiction and now you have trouble holding on to extra money. You might find yourself impulse-buying things you do not really need so you won't be tempted to spend money on drugs or alcohol. In such a case, you might end up living paycheck to paycheck and not have enough money for bills. Learning proper ways to handle and spend money is important in sobriety. Gambling is another money-related risk. Gambling brings a rush that can be similar to what your drug of choice brought to you. The thing is, gambling is not as easy as it seems. It puts most people into financial peril. People in these situations tend to keep gambling in hopes that they will hit the jackpot to help get them out of their hole, only to find themselves in worse debt. Just as drugs do, gambling can affect responsibilities and relationships. The difference between gambling and substance use is that gambling is more of a compulsion than a dependence. But it *is* connected to emotions, just like your addiction. If these emotions are not explored, then gambling can suck you in.

As you can see, drugs and alcohol are not the only things that can become addictive. Being aware is the best place to start. If you see a problem in another area, seek help through a counselor or other support group. And remember that there's a big difference between a problem and normal, natural behavior. Don't be afraid to do things you enjoy, such as shopping, having sex, or eating certain foods. This is one of those things that is not black or white; it's about balance. Balance might take time to figure out, but the important thing is to learn from your mistakes and not give up.

QUESTIONS

1. What are you concerned about when it comes to cross-addiction?

2. As research has shown, people who have worked or are working on addressing their issues in addiction tend to have a lower chance of cross-addiction. What are some current issues you are going through?

3. For you, what is a healthy approach to each of the following?
   - Alcohol
   - Food
   - Sex and pornography
   - Video games and technology
   - Money, shopping, and gambling

4. Look at your list above. Do you feel like you have another addiction? (It also could be something such as over-exercising, collecting certain items, drinking water, etc.)

5. If you are developing a cross-addiction, where can you seek help?

SECTION TWO

Addiction, Recovery, Change

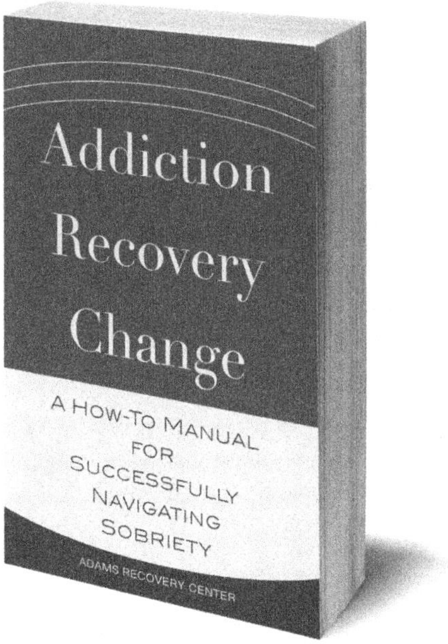

CHAPTER ONE

Setting Expectations after Treatment

In chapter one, we discuss that treatment does not solve all of someone's problems—sobriety is going to take work. On your journey, you will see who your sober supports are and who is waiting to see you fail. The reality is that life won't be picture-perfect after treatment. Treatment is the starting point for your new life, when you learn the basics such as being vulnerable and changing specific behaviors. You learn to step back and take a look at yourself.

When struggling with addiction, it is comforting to know there are others who have shared similar experiences. When you embrace others' experiences, you start learning to trust the process. The "process" is whatever fits the person working on sobriety. Some people view God as the process; some see the process as nature or the way the universe works. There is no right or wrong answer; it is simply what helps you move forward.

Once you've defined what the process means to you, you can reflect on why changing your environment is important but challenging. When you have been in addiction for months or years, you get comfortable with the way your life is going. But now, you need to look at people, places, or things that could get in the way of your sobriety. Remember: Not everyone wants to see you change for the better. Old people, places, and things go hand and hand with so-called "triggers." A trigger is something a person in recovery believes might lead him or her to use again. But in this chapter, you learn that triggers often are just excuses because you already want to use, and you actually have total control over how much power you give a trigger.

Before you leave treatment, we recommend you review what type of aftercare will work for you. There are Twelve-Step meetings such as Alcoholics Anonymous and Narcotics Anonymous, in addition to other support groups such as Secular Sobriety, Rational Recovery, or other nonaligned local groups. Support meetings are beneficial as long as you use them for the right reasons. Obsessing over attending multiple meetings instead of living your life is just substituting a new addictive pattern for an old one. Meetings also can be used as "hunting grounds." When you're new to sobriety, you need to take time to work on yourself. That means being careful about people who want to take advantage of you.

After treatment, explore your aftercare or intensive outpatient treatment options.

QUESTIONS

1. What will your life look like after treatment? Reflect on your sober supports, self-image, current struggles, etc.

2. The "process" can be many things. What does it mean to you?

3. When you look back on your life in active addiction, what are some people, places, and things you might need to avoid to remain sober? These can be people or things you identify as "triggers."

4. If things are not going to plan, what can you do to help your sobriety?

5. In Betty's story, she stated that entering treatment was one of the hardest things she had ever done. On her journey to sobriety, she learned to be different and not settle for the status quo. Write about your own experience entering treatment and how your sobriety is different from others' sobriety.

CHAPTER TWO

Finding Sober Supports

Finding sober support can be difficult when you are new to sobriety. Some people leave treatment with a lot of support, and some leave with none. This chapter reviews how beneficial sober support can be because, on your own, you cannot handle every situation life throws at you. It is okay to ask for help. Addiction has caused problems in almost every aspect of your life, and when things get hard, you start questioning yourself, which could lead to relapse.

The more sober support you have, the more likely you are to remain sober; however, some people get stuck in a belief that if a person has not struggled with addiction, then he or she cannot possibly understand someone in recovery. But that is not the case, and many excellent treatment professionals have no experience of addiction themselves—they simply want to help. That help consists of feedback or clarification as opposed to advice. Professionals are not there to solve your problems. In fact, not even your sober support can solve your problems. Only you have that power.

Jack's story reflects his journey to gaining sober support. When Jack entered treatment, he felt scared because he had nowhere to go and no one to lean on. Jack knew he wanted to stay away from old people, places, and things, but he was terrified that he was not strong enough. Jack worked with his treatment facility to find living arrangements and started to attend support meetings. Before Jack graduated treatment, he was more stable with his sober support.

QUESTIONS

1. Who are your sober supports? What characteristics do you need in a sober support?

2. What problems are you experiencing that you are willing to discuss with your sober support?

3. Is there anything you need from your sober support that you are not getting? Could you be honest and tell this person what you need?

4. Reflect on a time you were given advice and it was not helpful. What happened? Did you take the advice because it was someone else's idea, or did you come up with a solution on your own?

CHAPTER THREE

Assessing Your Relationships

When you assess your old relationships, you need to look at who would be quick to pull you back into the lifestyle of addiction. Misery loves company. So, look closely at people and what their intentions are. Do they want you to succeed, or do they want to bring you down? The latter are the people who would say, "Just do it one more time with me!" These people are also known as enablers, and they do not care about you having a substance issue. There are different types of enablers: those who are using, those who give in because you are difficult to deal with when you're using, and those who deal substances.

In Sam's story, you learn that he had his own house but it was not a healthy environment due to people in the house using. He could not kick them out because of the law, so he acted as though he had no other options. But by staying in this situation, he was putting his sobriety at risk. Sam discussed this situation with his counselor, and the counselor helped Sam see that he had options, even if they were unpleasant. Through processing, Sam realized he had a hard decision to make. In sobriety, you, too, are going to have hard decisions.

In life, you always have choices, even if you don't like those choices. All people tend to make choices based on what is comfortable, but breaking away from what is comfortable helps us grow. If you keep going back to the same things or the same lifestyle, nothing is going to change. When faced with a difficult decision, reflect on your active use.

QUESTIONS

1. Take an inventory of people in your life and ask these questions:
    - How many would not object to using with you again?

      ____

      ____

    - Are these people truly happy?

      ____

      ____

- Are they positive influences?

____

____

- Do they use, or are they recovering?

____

____

- What behaviors do they display?

____

____

2. Write about a time in your past when you were enabled. Did you manipulate the situation to be enabled? Who enabled you? Did you end up using?

____

____

____

____

____

3. In Sam's story, he was struggling with using friends and not having close sober support. He reported to his counselor that he did not have any other choices, but the truth was he had choices—he just did not like them. Describe a time when you had to choose among options you did not like.

____

____

____

____

4. If your home environment is not healthy, where else can you go? Make a list.

5. Now that you have reviewed your options, list the pros and cons for each one.

PROS	CONS

CHAPTER FOUR

Breaking Free of Codependence

Most people don't understand what codependency means. Codependency is defined as a relationship in which "two or more people have an excessive and unhealthy emotional and/or mental reliance on another person." Codependency is sometimes called "relationship addiction," and the relationships can be with anyone: parents, neighbors, friends, places of employment, etc. The list below breaks down some of the different characteristics of codependency:

- Believing you cannot exist without the other person: You must be around the other person all the time in order to function.
- Caregiving vs. partnership: The codependent person takes on a caregiver role instead of being an equal partner.
- Lack of emotional responsibility: Your emotions are determined by the other person. For example, "You being angry makes me angry."
- Rescuing: You feel like you can "save" or "fix" the other person.
- Lack of personal value: You relate being alone to failure, so you stay in an unhealthy relationship because it is "better" than being alone.
- Lack of assertiveness: You don't stand up for yourself because of the mind-set of, "I do not deserve a good relationship."
- People-pleasing: You make sure everyone else's needs are met before your own.
- Control issues: You find a way to control others for your own benefit.
- Obsessive thinking: You take your thoughts, feelings, and actions to the extreme. For example, you might think your partner is cheating on you simply because he or she is not in your presence.
- Low self-esteem: You find low or no value in yourself as a human.
- Exaggeration of perceived failure and mistakes: You feel any mistake is a failure. This is connected with all-or-nothing thinking.

If you find yourself displaying these characteristics, then it's time to do some evaluating. You might not have to end these relationships, but you do need to repair them, perhaps by attending counseling and working on setting boundaries. You also might need to focus on yourself. In codependent relationships, you focus a lot on the other person and lose who you really are. Putting the focus back on you does not make you self-centered or selfish; it allows you time to reflect on your own thoughts and feelings.

After you figure out those thoughts and feelings, you need to take ownership of things you cannot control. Understand that you are not responsible for what other people think or feel. You cannot make anyone feel sad, mad, happy, etc. People manage their own feelings and make their own decisions. Your

words and/or actions might have an impact, but other people are responsible for themselves, just like you are responsible for yourself.

If you decide to move on from a codependent relationship, be aware of the struggle that might come with this action. Codependent people will do or say anything to keep you in their lives, but stand strong and do not be sucked back in. You might feel guilty, but keep in mind you are making choices to improve yourself.

You are responsible only for how *you* live *your* life. To help you follow through living your life, it is okay to seek help from professionals, sober support, and support meetings.

QUESTIONS

1. In your own words, what is codependency? Do you think you are in a codependent relationship or relationships? If so, with whom?

____

____

____

____

____

2. What characteristics define your codependent relationship(s)? Provide specific examples.

____

____

____

____

____

3. Take some time to reflect and get to know yourself, independent of anyone else. What are things you like or enjoy vs. things you don't like and don't enjoy?
   - Likes:

   - Dislikes:

4. If you are choosing to end a codependent relationship, what can you say to stand your ground? Example: "I understand that this upsets you, but I am doing this for me." How do you think the conversation will go?

5. When you are in a codependent relationship and you need assistance—whether you are ending the relationship or you need to set boundaries—where can you go and from whom can you seek help?

CHAPTER FIVE

Battling Boredom

Being bored is among the top reasons why people relapse. Many people start using drugs because they cannot stand their life to one degree or another. When entering sobriety, you are identifying sober support, working on yourself, and distancing yourself from toxic relationships—but through all of that, you will still find time to be bored. Boredom is connected to restlessness, and when restlessness gets intense, we're tempted to put all our energy into something—which could backfire. The example in the chapter describes a person going through grief and then distracting himself from feeling any emotions by staying busy. That's not a healthy way to cope; it's better to take time to go over your thoughts and feelings to address them productively.

When it comes to boredom and sobriety, balance is key. You cannot take a break from life, nor should you overdo it. Even putting too much time into treatment can be dangerous. Boredom is part of the transition into sobriety. In early sobriety, you need to discover what healthy activities will keep you involved in your own life. As the book advises, "You should spend time feeding your soul, not your habit." Boredom can bring on feelings of anxiety or depression. Such feelings are normal when you are not sure what your next move should be, so try to see boredom as an opportunity to learn more about yourself.

Boredom can be perceived as a negative, but it's actually the byproduct of being free. You are free to explore things you could or would not do while under the influence. Reflect on how much time was wasted on your active addiction: finding the drug, getting the money, finding your dealer, finding a place to use, getting high, and then recovering—only to complete the cycle again. Were you really living?

QUESTIONS

1. What would be a sign you are overdoing something to distract yourself from reflecting on your thoughts and feelings? **An example:** Two weeks ago, I found out my best friend passed away. Instead of dealing with the grief, I decided to attend three support meetings daily, and I have been doing this for two weeks. By attending multiple meetings, I am distracting myself from the real problem.

2. What feelings do you experience when you get bored?

3. What activities do you enjoy or would you like to try? With whom can you do these activities?

4. Sobriety comes with freedom. What joy has sobriety brought to your life?

5. When you look in the mirror, whom do you see? Reflect on the type of person you were when you were using versus the person you are today. Describe the positive growth in yourself.

CHAPTER SIX

Encountering Temptation

Understanding that you have an addiction is key to understanding this chapter. No matter where you go or whom you are around, your addiction does not go away—it simply gets easier to handle. This can be a good thing or a bad thing. Some people in treatment develop an overly confident attitude and think they can go back around old people, places, and things without relapsing. This might be true for some, but we do not recommend it. To fight temptation, we strongly advise you to not put yourself in a situation that could tempt you.

That being said, it's important to remember that "triggers" are really just excuses. Something like a beer bottle, for example, cannot make you drink. The bottle doesn't have any power or control over you unless you allow it to. Supposed triggers can be anything and can be everywhere, but you cannot make them a reason to stop living your life. Taking a trigger and looking at it for what it is can be empowering. And for every excuse you have to use again, you can find ten reasons you will *not* use again.

Sometimes when clients leave treatment, they start to think they are "cured." This mind-set is dangerous and could lead you to use drugs/alcohol again just to test your limits. This goes hand in hand with the one-more-time mentality of "I can use it just once." This attitude does not need to relate only to your drug of choice; it can connect to possible substitution, as well, when you're experimenting with or using another drug besides your drug of choice. This behavior is also dangerous. If this is something you start to experience, then you might want to look at why you still feel the need to escape from your thoughts and feelings. If you're reverting to your previous behaviors, you probably need to look at your core issues and why you started using in the first place.

QUESTIONS

1. What excuses or so-called "triggers" are you allowing to have power over your life? What can you do to adjust your thinking?

____

____

____

____

____

2. List ten reasons why you want to stay sober.

3. Do you think that one day you will be able to use drugs and alcohol again? Why or why not? What are your thoughts about the idea that another substance could lead you back to your drug of choice?

4. What were your thoughts about your addiction prior to entering treatment?

5. Why do you think you started using substances? These answers can relate to your core issues (for example: difficult childhood, being molested/raped, domestic violence, codependency, lack of emotional regulation, etc.). There is no right or wrong answer.

6. In Rich's story, Rich blamed everyone else for his problems and for him drinking so much. Toward the end, Rich started taking responsibility for his own actions. What are you willing to take responsibility for?

CHAPTER SEVEN

Common Questions and Thinking Errors

Treatment is not meant to "fix" or "cure" you; in fact, nothing will fix or cure you. Addiction is a daily struggle. Substance abuse is a behavioral disorder, and behavioral disorders are not curable. But, they are treatable as long as you are actively working on your sobriety. When actively working your program, you will see the problematic behaviors diminish over time.

When struggling with addiction, some people take the route of having medication-assisted treatment (MAT), which could include methadone, Suboxone, or Vivitrol. These medications, when taken as prescribed, help with opiate withdrawal. These medications will not cure you, but they will help reduce physical discomfort and make it easier to focus on recovery. When it comes to your health, it is important to seek medical attention for any health problems, substance-related or not.

There are a lot of opinions when it comes to addiction. Some people think "relapse is a part of recovery," while some say, "You will abuse substances again and there's nothing you can do about it." These are examples of black-and-white or all-or-nothing thinking. When people say things like this to you, they could be projecting: recalling their own experience and relating it to you. For example, "I relapsed, so you will relapse."

This comes back to the idea of failing vs. making a mistake. The truth is you might use again, but that only indicates that your coping skills were not strong enough. That's a fixable situation—not a failure. You need to remember that you're human, and humans make mistakes and give into temptation from time to time.

The idea of "relapse," however, has failure built into it. If you expect to relapse, then you're just waiting to fail—or giving yourself an excuse to use again. There's a difference between accepting one's human foibles and rationalizing or justifying substance abuse by saying, "Well, I'm only human." If you do find yourself drawn back into a lifestyle of using, you need to look deeper into yourself and figure out what is drawing you down that path again.

You might or might not know why you abuse substances. The important thing is that if you've learned a behavior, you can unlearn it. You have the ability and the power to change. You have the choice about what path you take.

QUESTIONS

1. What do you think about medication-assisted treatment?

2. How do you view success and failure?

3. Are you being tempted by your old lifestyle? If you were to go back, what could be some consequences?

4. What behaviors do you need to unlearn?

SECTION
THREE

Assess, Rebuild, Connect

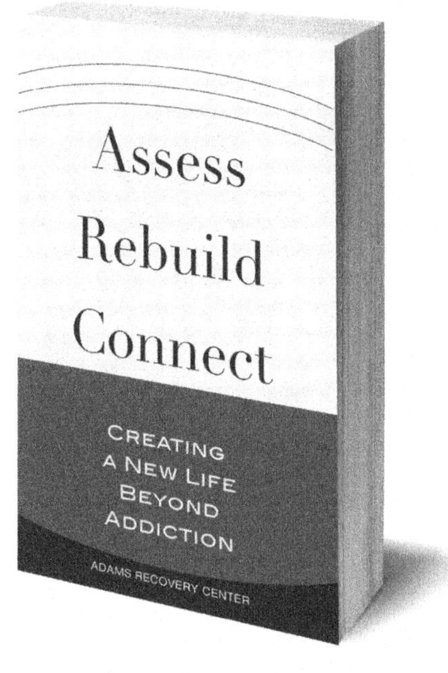

CHAPTER ONE

A Quick Overview

This chapter summarizes the key topics from books one and two to prepare readers to get the most out of *Assess, Rebuild, Connect.*

First and foremost, it's helpful to understand addiction as a physical and mental dependence on something. And what's more, dealing with that addiction will be a lifelong process. There's no shame or weakness in that; it's just something you have to stay on top of as you would any health or medical issue.

Even once you're clean, your underlying issues will remain to some degree. In fact, as you work through the process of healing, you might even uncover new problems. That's completely normal, though, and is a natural part of getting and staying clean and sober. A good analogy is keeping a car running smoothly. As any car owner knows, there are always maintenance issues, whether it's a simple oil change or a major transmission problem. Be as willing to care for yourself as you are to care for your car.

All of that maintenance is part of trusting the process. You'll hear about that concept a lot, because it's such a crucial piece of recovery. Recovery—whether early on or decades later—will never be easy, because life isn't easy for anyone. The trials and tribulations you experience are part of "the process," and you have to trust that life is worth living and fighting for even when times are tough. The low moments are lessons that make you stronger for whatever comes next. When you stop trying to control everything, you become more able to grow and develop.

Setting realistic expectations also will help you stay positive and more able to make healthy decisions. In sobriety, life won't be perfect all the time. You'll experience boredom at times, and you'll have moments of wondering whether you'll be able to accomplish your goals and feel like you're making progress. Again, all of this anxiety and self-doubt is totally normal. Remember to think of your new life as an opportunity to learn more about yourself and develop new interests and passions that fill your spare time and keep you engaged in life.

Once you embrace this new chapter in your life, anything is possible for you. The sky is the limit!

QUESTIONS

1. When you think of addiction as a lifelong process, how do you feel? Is there any comfort you take in knowing you don't have to have all the answers right away?

2. How do you feel about the idea that things always work out as they should?

3. So far, how has your recovery process compared to your expectations for it? Has anything been better than you anticipated?

CHAPTER TWO

Rebuilding Trust

Trust is something with which many people struggle when they're new to sobriety. You might have trouble figuring out how and whom to trust. You also might struggle to regain the trust of others. During active addiction, you probably broke the trust of loved ones but gained the trust of other active users. You learned to trust that your drug dealer was giving you the "good stuff," and you trusted that your using friends would hook you up if you were out of money. But now you want and need relationships built on real trust and healthy habits, and it's important to explore how you relate to trust in general. Was there trust in your family when you were young? Was your trust broken by someone close to you? As you answer questions like this, you will become able to build trust again.

You can trust someone for different reasons. It could be that the person is non-judgmental, he is caring, or she's achieved long-term sobriety. You do not need to grant everyone the same level of trust. You might entrust your biggest secret to your best friend but not share the same secret in a sober-support meeting such as AA or NA. When you do decide to share information, you are doing so for your own benefit. You are reaching out to help yourself and not to meet the needs of others.

Another big part of trusting others is following your gut feeling. If you think you cannot trust someone, then listen to your gut. Trusting yourself and your instinct can go a long way. Your instincts might have gotten you into trouble in the past, but just as you are changing, so are your instincts. You might be asking yourself, "If no one can trust me, then how can I possibly trust myself?" The fact is, you can. It can help to repeat mantras such as "I am trustworthy" or "I can be trusted." This might seem silly, but it works if you follow through with it. People in your life are going to remind you that you have broken their trust in the past, but you need to keep moving forward because you are learning to be a new, trustworthy person.

When trust is broken, emotions such as anger, resentment, and hostility come into play. These can be worked through in a variety of ways. It is important to speak the truth and be honest with all parties, and your words and behaviors need to match. You can communicate honestly through a phone call, in a letter, or face to face. Make sure you are talking not only about your struggles but about the good things you are experiencing as well. With honesty, we encourage you to set boundaries. Boundaries help show your loved ones that you are still moving forward in your sobriety. You might inform your family what parts of your sobriety you are willing to share and what parts you need to keep private. When you do this, your family might not believe you. When earning trust, you need to be a little open-minded and flexible while upholding your boundaries. You might need to have a family member drive you to a meeting instead of you borrowing the car, or you might need to volunteer to take a home drug test. These are actions that help build trust with someone.

Also, you are going to want to start clean with everyone. This means no longer having contact with dealers or "friends" you used with, because none of those people are going to respect your boundaries. If you continue to communicate with people from your active use, your family might have a harder time wanting to build trust with you. Be honest, and trust will come—not overnight, but in the time it needs.

QUESTIONS

1. How has trust played out in your life? How did you grow up? Have you been to jail? Do you have trust with people in authority?

2. Whom do you trust? Whom do you not trust? Explain why you do or do not have trust with these people.

3. Do you trust yourself or your instincts? If not, how can you improve in this area?

4. What do you need to be honest about?

5. What are boundaries you would like to put in place to help build trust?

6. With whom do you need to stop communicating?

CHAPTER THREE

Living with Integrity

Treatment is not just about changing behaviors; it is about changing your character and building integrity. What is integrity? Integrity is connected to honesty and morality—your values. So, ask yourself: Are you doing the right thing even when no one is watching? Are you following rules and laws? Are you being honest? As you grow in integrity, you become more open and willing to listen to others, to follow up on self-reflection, and to apply what you have learned.

These questions can help you evaluate whether you are living with integrity:

- Are you meeting your goals and following through on your commitments?
- Are you being open and honest with your family about your current situation? If you are struggling, are you telling them or hiding it from them?
- Are you lashing out at others and then pretending everything is fine?

Being honest is the key! If you are lying to friends or family, you are lying to yourself. Sometimes it's by telling an untruth; other times, it's through a lie of omission. An example of this would be if your mom asks, "Are you doing heroin again?" and you say "no" but leave out the fact that you used cocaine the day before. Part of living with integrity and honesty is caring about those around you, whether they are close family members or strangers walking down the street.

Open communication also ties in to integrity. Asking questions of others can help you figure out how well you are actually doing in your sobriety. Questions create a dialogue that can help you improve in areas where you could be struggling. Being open and honest is contagious and can make you a positive role model. This helps not only you but others around you. It is important to think about whom you are associating with. If you are hanging around people who are dishonest, then you are going to start making excuses for them, which connects you to their lies. If you are connected to a lie, how can you practice integrity? The fact is, you can't.

You will hear that balance is basically the number one thing in sobriety. Creating balance in your life means saying no sometimes, even when it's hard. You might feel guilty at first, but think about this: If you overcommit yourself and then fail to do what you've agreed to do, you're not living with integrity. When you're new to sobriety, you feel the need to say yes to help make up for lost time. But if you say yes to everything, you find that your schedule is jammed with events and there is no time for yourself or for focusing on your sobriety. This is why balance is so important. When trying to find balance, you will see that you are not perfect. That is where humility comes into play. Being humble helps not only you but others as well. If you make a mistake and share about it, it can help someone else grow from his or her own mistakes. Being humble teaches us that failures can lead to success. Making mistakes and learning from them only builds your integrity.

QUESTIONS

1. How do you demonstrate integrity? Think about these questions:
   - Are you meeting your goals and following through on your commitments?

   - Are you being open and honest with your family about your current situation? If you are struggling, are you telling them or hiding it from them?

   - Are you lashing out at others and then pretending everything is fine?

2. What does it mean to you to be honest? Are you being honest? Do you need to come clean about a lie?

3. What does open communication look like in your life? Discuss communication with yourself, your family, and other people.

4. Describe a time when you made a mistake. How did you grow from it? How can you share your story?

CHAPTER FOUR

Navigating New Firsts

You've experienced a lot of firsts in your life, even many you don't remember. Most of them are accompanied by feelings of fear, anxiety, or excitement, whether by you or your parents and loved ones.

Getting sober brings about a whole host of first-time experiences that create similar feelings. In sobriety, you are entering a new world with a new mind-set. You could be parenting without substances for the first time, going to your first family event sober, or having sober sex for the first time. Any first can create an emotional reaction that can affect your self-esteem. For example, think about when you first stopped using; you probably felt panicked knowing you no longer had a way to numb your thoughts and feelings.

The first time you do anything, you are exploring the unknown, which creates a sense of discomfort. There is a saying: To get comfortable, you have to get *un*comfortable. This is not easy, because change is hard. In sobriety, you will see that not everything is carefree and easy but that you *can* learn to do things differently without drugs and alcohol. With change, you need to keep an open mind and remind yourself why making a change is important to you. To help deal with your emotions during unstable times, break down what you are going through. Use this process:

- Analyze each issue or event. Why is it important?
- Explore why there is anxiety or fear attached to the issue. Is what you are feeling based on current facts or a past experience?
- Set smaller goals to help minimize the emotional load.

When you break down your emotions and understand what is going on, it is easier to find a resolution. Otherwise, feeling overwhelmed can paralyze you. To stay on track, it is important to acknowledge your strengths and weaknesses and understand how they affect your sobriety. Remember: Maintaining your sobriety is your number one priority.

Emotions can run particularly high when you're beginning or ending a relationship. New relationships bring fear, vulnerability, anticipation, and excitement. When starting a new relationship, you have to understand your motives. Relationships are complicated, and if you are not the best you, it might create a downward spiral. Think about everything you have going on, such as working, attending meetings, making amends with family and friends, and still making time for self-care. Do you have time and energy to invest into someone else? Are you entering a relationship to avoid something else? Starting a new relationship could bring back memories from past relationships, which can create self-doubt or resentment. For instance, when going out on a date for the first time, you might think you are not going to be fun or you won't be able to open up without drinking or using drugs. These self-defeating thoughts can increase the chance of relapse. To figure out if you are ready for a relationship, ask yourself these questions:

- Why am I considering getting involved in an intimate relationship at this time?
- Am I creating a diversion because I am overwhelmed by other areas of my life?
- Am I able to commit to another person's wants and needs while still caring for my own?
- How well balanced are the other areas of my life?

Once you figure out your answers to these questions, you can take the next steps to set goals and work on how to achieve those goals. If you cannot manage another responsibility, such as a relationship, then consider waiting until you have more time and energy to give a relationship what it needs to succeed. Give yourself the correct amount of time for *you*. Everyone's timing for building a relationship is different. You are still growing and learning about who you are sober.

That brings us back to ending relationships. There are some people in your life who are not positive role models and might not want you to continue your journey toward sobriety. Even when you need to end these relationships because you know they are toxic, you might still feel an emotional fear that takes over. If the relationship is toxic, then why is it hard to move on from it? The answer relates to being comfortable. Think about these questions:

- Are you holding on to a bad relationship to have something that is familiar?
- Are you unsure how to create a new relationship if you let one go?
- By staying in a toxic relationship, are you really facing your fears?
- How can you grow in recovery if you are unwilling to let go of people?

Once you figure out your thoughts and feelings, you can allow yourself to set goals to move forward.

The first time you do something, embrace it! If it does not go as planned, then learn from it and try again.

QUESTIONS

1. What are some "firsts" you are going to experience in sobriety? What emotions do you feel about these events? How can you manage your uncomfortable emotions?

2. Why is changing important to you? What new behaviors do you need to adopt to maintain your sobriety?

3. What changes are you experiencing that bring about a feeling of being overwhelmed or anxious?

4. What relationship do you need to end? How do you plan on doing this? What concerns you about doing this?

CHAPTER FIVE

Avoiding Becoming Overwhelmed

The feeling of being overwhelmed is a natural part of sobriety, but if it is not managed, you could end up right back where you started: in addiction. When you're in treatment, you might start to realize how much you missed during addiction. You want to make up for lost time by getting a job, spending time with your children, reconnecting with loved ones, etc. This can get exhausting pretty quickly! Remember, the key is balance. To maintain balance, consider getting a planner and writing down a daily schedule. In that schedule, make sure there is time for *you*. If you are not leaving enough time for self-care, you could be putting your sobriety on the back burner.

Most people who experience the feeling of being overwhelmed forget to ask for help. In sobriety, you might think you have to be independent and that asking for help diminishes that. The truth is it doesn't. Asking for help is a humbling thing, and most people are afraid to do it. They are afraid of the negative response they might get. They also might perceive asking for help as showing weakness. But asking for help does not make you a failure; it makes you human. When you are feeling down, alone, stressed, or overwhelmed, reach out for help. You are not a superhero!

Being a perfectionist also leads to the feeling of being overwhelmed. Many, if not most, of us have been programmed for perfectionism since we were children. You might have tried to be the best soccer player on the field or the best actress in the school play. If you missed a goal or forgot one of your lines, you might have thought, "I will never be good enough." Everyone, including you, wants to reach his or her full potential in life. But there's a way to do that without dwelling on negatives. Instead, ask yourself these questions:

1. Did you give your best effort in the task?
2. Did you consider the interests of others and yourself?
3. Did you procrastinate?
4. Are your expectations realistic?

Your answers to these questions should reflect someone who shows empathy, sets realistic goals, has managed time wisely, and has given a genuine effort. If your answers do not reflect this, then you can now take a step and make a change. Remember, no one is perfect no matter how much success he or she has.

Like perfectionism, procrastination can be dangerous to your recovery. Putting off something to the last minute sets you up for failure. In addiction, you probably procrastinated a lot. For example, you might have said something like, "I will go to treatment Monday. But for now, I am going to enjoy the weekend." Procrastination isn't so different in sobriety. If you are putting off things such as meetings, doctor appointments, college registration, etc., then try to identify why you don't want to follow through with the things you need to get done. What's the root issue you need to address? Everyone needs a day off every now and

then. Just make sure you hold yourself accountable and get right back into your routine after your day of R&R.

Feeling overwhelmed is going to happen at some point in your sobriety, and that is normal. The key is to make sure you know healthy ways to manage it. Step one is learning to say no, which is easier said than done. Saying no allows others to know you have boundaries and that you are focused on yourself. It is okay to help others if you have the time, but if you have limited time, it is not a good idea to take on more. Step two is making sure you are eating a healthful diet and getting enough sleep. Maintaining a routine will help keep these things stable. Eat breakfast, lunch, and dinner at the same times every day and allow yourself enough time to fall asleep without interruption. Step three is finding time to embrace some peace and quiet. For your mental health, it is encouraged to find twenty minutes a day without TV, video games, music, or other interruptions. The quiet time allows your brain to relax and unwind. When you are relaxed, you can keep an open mind and work on dealing with your emotions in a healthful manner.

QUESTIONS

1. Make yourself a daily schedule. You can use the one provided or make your own.

TODAY'S TASKS | DATE ________________

TIME	TASK DESCRIPTION

2. Make a list of people you feel comfortable asking for help. Why do you feel comfortable reaching out to these individuals?

3. In what ways are you a perfectionist? Have you experienced the feeling of being overwhelmed by this behavior? How can you change it?

4. Was there a time in your active addiction when you procrastinated on something? Are you still procrastinating now? What are you not following through with and why? Explain the emotions connected to your behavior.

5. Reflect on the schedule you made in item one. Do you have too much on your plate, or do you need to find more things to do? Think about the following: Is there enough time for you? Is there enough family time? Is there enough time for meetings and working on your sobriety? Are you getting enough sleep? Have you built in meal times? Make changes as needed and describe your thought process in making those changes.

CHAPTER SIX

Managing Family Dynamics

Now that you are sober, you might be thinking you want to go back to the person you used to be before your addiction, or your family might want the "old you" back. That's a destructive thought process. When you think about yourself prior to addiction, were you happy? What were the issues that led to your addiction? If you were to go back to who you once were, you might end up back in the same spot. On page 65 of *Assess, Rebuild, Connect* it states, "To move forward, there can be no going back."

Now that you are moving forward as a new person, family dynamics are going to change. Your addiction changed you, and it changed how you interacted with others; trust has been broken, communication has been compromised, and a few family members might be in denial. Families are all different and unique. Some families share everything, while others find it best to keep issues private. Whatever type of family you come from, you might feel the need to protect your loved ones due to the guilt and shame you put them through. Or, you might blame yourself for all the dysfunction you created. The same can go for family members. Some family might try to defend your actions or blame others for your struggles with addiction. In any case, communication has been affected, and it needs to be improved.

Improving communication, of course, isn't easy. You're likely to face arguments, raised voices, and hurt feelings. One challenge when it comes to communication is feeling fear about how someone else will respond, in addition to frustration with not feeling heard. Another challenge is that a lot of people do not want to open up to discuss their struggles or a family member's struggles with addiction. Addiction comes with judgment and labeling, which makes people want to shut down and ignore it. This brings up denial. When you cover up someone's addiction, you are not allowing communication the opportunity to change or develop. You have to accept there is a problem before you can find a solution.

Communication has two key components: trust and empathy. Your family members or loved ones might have a hard time with trust and empathy due to the things you have put them through. The thing to remember is that trust and empathy go both ways. You need to trust that your family is not going to enable your negative behaviors. A loved one needs to trust that you are going to follow through and do the right things for yourself and your sobriety. Rebuilding trust will take time.

When it comes to empathy, a lot of people do not understand that it is different from sympathy. Sympathy is defined as feeling sorry for someone. When a family member is sympathetic, he or she is enabling an addict. But when someone has empathy, he or she understands what someone is going through. Using positive encouragement and enforcement can help someone make the right decision on their own. As long as you work together, trust and empathy can improve the communication in the relationship.

When a loved one watches an addict struggle, sometimes she might fantasize about a "better life"—a life in which she would no longer need to worry or a life in which the addict no longer feels pain. This is connected to the loss of hope. This does not mean the loved one has given up on the addicted person; it just means she is frustrated, overwhelmed, and not sure what else to do. When family members feel like they have no more options, effective communication and setting boundaries can be helpful tools. (See pages 70-72.) In the example from *Assess, Rebuild, Connect,* you can see how communication can be twisted and unclear; you also can see how important it can be when done effectively.

To help bring change, you need to understand the difference between healthy and unhealthy boundaries. Boundaries are not a punishment. They need to be clear and defined to serve both parties, and if a boundary is broken, there has to be follow-through with consequences. If you set boundaries but don't enforce them, people will walk all over you.

With all the changes that come in sobriety, it is important that you continue to put in the work and educate yourself, along with loved ones. You're going to face many emotions that you are going to need to process, but don't dwell on them.

Effective communication works best when both parties are on the same page. Take time to sit down with an open mind, no distractions, and prepare yourself for what you want to say or what you plan on accomplishing during the conversation. Be sure to use "I" statements. Examples would be, "I feel upset when I see this..." or "I worry when..." This allows you to take ownership and not place blame. When you start a conversation with "You did this..." or "When you do that..." it sends an aggressive message. Other things to think about are body language and tone of voice. Sometimes it is not what you say, but it is how you say it. When you have a conversation with your arms crossed and eyes rolling, it gives the message that you are not listening or you are becoming defensive.

In a perfect world, there would be no arguments, but that is not the case. Everyone has his or her own perceptions. Just know it is okay to disagree and you are not going to win every disagreement you have. When using communication in a healthy manner, both parties should feel safe, accepted, and understood.

Reconnecting with someone in sobriety can be challenging, but with healthy communication and boundaries, you both can move forward. Do not give up hope.

QUESTIONS

1. What type of family do you have? Is your family open and honest, or do they keep everything secret and quiet?

2. What challenges do you face when communicating with family members or loved ones?

3. How have you displayed sympathy and empathy in your life? This can be while sober or under the influence.

4. Explain a time you experienced struggles with communicating effectively. Think about the message you received. What message were you probably supposed to receive, and what was your response? (Tone of voice and body language play a part in this.)

5. Make a list of boundaries you need to put in place and what the consequences are if those boundaries are broken.

6. Practice using "I" statements. Write down or role-play things you can say to help others understand your current struggles.

CHAPTER SEVEN

Handling the Holidays

Holidays are meant to bring families and friends together to celebrate, but for someone in recovery, holidays can be difficult. When coming together, you could experience stress, conflicts with individuals, and temptation. Also, your past might come up, which can be quite uncomfortable. Despite these potential challenges, you can learn healthy ways to survive the holidays.

In chapter five, you learned that making a schedule is important. Sticking to a schedule helps you limit the amount of down time you have, which gives you less time to think about using. Holidays, of course, interrupt our daily schedules, which can lead to a feeling of being off balance. For example, when holidays roll around, a lot of businesses are closed or have half days. If you have this extra time off work, you could become bored, which can lead to using again. Even when your schedule is altered, try to stick to it as closely as possible. Wake up at the same time, eat a healthy breakfast, practice some self-care, and add a sober activity. By doing these things, you can keep something of a "normal" routine.

Holidays can bring on different emotions, both good and bad. They also can bring up the past. You might attend an event where someone special is not there because he has passed away or because she is not someone you can have in your life in sobriety. It can be hard to face the holidays knowing this special person is not there, and as a result, you might mask your true emotions to keep everyone around you happy for the celebration. Grieving during this time can be challenging because your emotions are running higher than normal. When this happens, you might start to justify that one drink or one more use will be okay. Instead of taking this route, utilize your healthy coping skills; reach out to speak to someone, go to a meeting, use breathing techniques, etc.

The reason holidays are emotional is due to the expectations you place on yourself or others. You might think you need to bring the best gift because you haven't been there for the last three years, or you might be expected to act a certain way to make others feel more comfortable ("wearing a mask"). Expectations can cause self-defeating thoughts and create resentments in the long run. That can lead to guilt and shame, making it easy to slip into a relapse. Your main focus should be your sobriety. If you think anything will get in the way of that, you might need to make other plans. You could ask someone to go to lunch the next day to avoid a crowded family event. If this person is supportive of your sobriety, he or she will understand.

Try to remember that a holiday is just another day. Use your coping skills to help in the moment. Things will slow down soon and you will get back into your daily routine.

Family members can be hard to deal with at the holidays. Some people you haven't seen in a while, and others you might not want to see but have to. In these situations, you might find yourself making small talk, which can be difficult. When families or friends get together, they generally are talking and drinking,

and conversations can switch to become negative. Try to stay away from the family drama. If you know this happens at your family gatherings, then you need to go into an event with a plan. Maybe you can bring your "accountabili-buddy," a friend who understands what you are going through. This person can help hold you accountable and can assist if a situation gets sticky.

One of the biggest holidays that brings up anxiety is New Year's Eve. We tend to end up pondering our pasts and our futures. You might think about the previous year and everything you did not accomplish. You could also experience fear from looking into your future. Holidays bring on many emotions, so it can be helpful to think about the purpose of the holiday. New Year's is a time to start over, and that is what you are doing in your sobriety. You can survive the holidays as long as you use your healthy coping skills.

QUESTIONS

1. If your schedule gets interrupted by the holidays, what are some things you can do to keep you from boredom?

2. What makes you uncomfortable around the holidays?

3. What are some things you can say to others if you cannot attend a holiday celebration?

4. Who could be your "accountabili-buddy"? What could be your plan if you need help getting out of a situation?

5. What emotions do you feel when you think of New Year's? What are some goals you want to bring into the next new year?

CHAPTER EIGHT

Connecting to Your Passion

Having a passion in your life can help you stay on the path of sobriety, and recovery gives you the chance to find that passion by trying new things and growing outside your comfort zone. As a child, you probably had lots of passions and interests, and you weren't afraid to go after them. But as we age, we all have a tendency to worry more about risk and failure and get bogged down in our daily responsibilities. In addiction, drug use takes over everything. You leave your passions behind and focus solely on using.

In recovery, you can chase your passion the way you once chased your drug of choice. In your drug use, all your time and energy went to getting money to acquire your drug, finding your dealer, buying your drug, using it, and starting the cycle again. Now that you are sober, you can put your resources into something positive. You have the ability, and the responsibility, to set and pursue your own dreams and goals. Everyone finds happiness in different places, and you are the only person who can make yourself happy.

When finding a new passion, it's important to keep an open mind. Your passion does not need to be huge or life-altering. In fact, it's best to start with something small so as not to become overwhelmed. For example, try one new thing or introduce yourself to a new person. Trying new things can be scary because we can't predict the outcome. Will you enjoy the new thing? Will you be good at it? Who knows! The problem with fear is that it sets limitations for the future. You've probably said or heard things along the lines of "I am too old to do that" or "I missed my chance." But these statements can keep you in your negative mind-set; they don't help you foster new beginnings. When you live a passionless life, you might experience resentments or regret—even guilt and shame. When you have a passion, you have a life. You're not just going through the motions.

A passion does not need to become a life-long career. Think of a passion as a hobby, doing something you love. Individuals who are just existing tend to be more complacent and experience more boredom, which can lead to using drugs to escape from the daily routine.

When you were a child, your passions changed frequently. Maybe at first you loved to ride your bike every day, but later you preferred to read or play an instrument. Even as an adult you will go through a trial-and-error phase. You might try something like an exercise class and realize you enjoy cooking classes more. Or, you might sign up for a twelve-week glass-blowing class and love it, but it is available only once a year. In that case, you might need to find another hobby to keep you from experiencing boredom the rest of the time.

It is important that you do not become fixated on one hobby or goal to avoid becoming frustrated and having self-defeating thoughts that could make you want to quit. Goals need to be realistic—not easy, just realistic. Challenges can be good for you and can help you continue to grow. If you find yourself

struggling, think of *ERR!* This stands for Escape, Relax, Reward, and it allows you to scream it out, shake it off, and continue to move forward.

No matter what you choose to pursue in sobriety, remember what passion is really all about: bringing you joy and helping you become a better you.

QUESTIONS

1. What was your passion as a child?

2. What are your passions/hobbies now that you are an adult?

3. Are your hobbies/passions short-term or longer-term goals? How can you work on achieving these goals? Make a plan.

4. What are some ways you *ERR* (Escape, Relax, and Reward)?)

CHAPTER NINE

Medical Care and the Importance of Healthy Thinking

Researchers and physicians have recognized that the mind and body are connected, but many people do not believe or understand that their mental well-being could be the cause of physical health issues. Having a healthy mind is a crucial component to healthy living. When your mind is clear and refreshed, you will notice it has an impact on your mood and, often, on how you feel physically. If you are holding on to negativity, then you will notice the physical toll it takes on your body. If you are open-minded and relaxed, you might notice you have more energy, motivation, and focus. The mind and body create a circle; if you are complaining about your discomfort physically, then you might start to develop self-pity, which leads to depression, which can lead to more self-pity and discomfort. A holistic view of emotional, mental, and physical health is vital to starting and maintaining sobriety.

While in treatment, you should have multiple medical assessments to see how you are progressing and changing. This is your opportunity to advocate for yourself to make sure you are getting what you need mentally, emotionally, and physically. Part of this process is learning to make good decisions on your own, because once you leave treatment, no one will be there to hold your hand or hold you accountable. To assess your progress, ask yourself these questions:

- Am I advocating for my own health care?
- Am I accurately assessing my pain? Or am I catastrophizing my symptoms?
- If I am exaggerating these symptoms, am I seeking immediate relief?
- Have I assessed how seeking immediate relief might jeopardize my sobriety?
- How receptive am I to instruction, guidance, and education?
- Overall, what is my level of receptivity?

Research is still being done on the mind and body, but it already has been found that forgiveness can lower the chances of heart attack by improving cholesterol levels and sleep and reducing pain, anxiety, depression, and stress. When you forgive things you have done or that have been done to you, your mood and emotions begin to change. After taking away the drugs and alcohol, you might find that evaluating your emotions is harder than you thought.

Sobriety gives you a different view of the world, and you have to learn the proper skills to navigate your new life. You have to make different decisions than you did in your active use. Part of this involves learning not to rely on over-the-counter (OTC) drugs.

OTC medications can be dangerous to someone in sobriety because they can be used as a crutch, the first step down a slippery slope that can lead back to your drug of choice. When you are new to sobriety, OTC medication can be used to help numb pain you are feeling. Most people think OTC substances are

harmless, but that is not the truth. Relying on OTC medications could drive you back to your old thinking and negative behaviors. The medications might work temporarily, but eventually they will not provide the same effect and you will seek something stronger. There are ways to address your health issues without using OTC drugs, such as drinking more water. For example, staying hydrated can help "cure" a headache.

It's important to understand that pain is a part of life. Pain is not a bad thing, and that is something a lot of people don't grasp. If you think pain should not be in your life, then you are headed down a path of sabotaging your recovery. Pain helps us grow and develop. When you experience pain in your body, it's your body trying to tell you there could be a bigger problem. Masking your pain only keeps you stuck and unable to move forward. You allow yourself to stay in a vicious cycle, only to experience more or different pain.

When it comes to pain and medical personnel, you might find yourself unable to trust that they have your best interest at heart. Since you have been self-medicating, you believe there is no way someone else can help you. But look back on your addiction. You endured a lot of stress without realizing it. You probably lied, snuck around, stole things, and tried your best to hide your addiction. All of that can add to your stress level, which affects you mentally and physically. The chapter references a book, *The Mind-Gut Connection*, which discusses how hormones are connected to mental illness, anxiety disorders, panic attacks, and depression. The book also discusses stress-sensitive physical disorders such as obesity, metabolic syndrome, heart attacks, and strokes. Finding healthy and proper coping skills can help reduce stress and other mental health concerns.

Sobriety is different for everyone. Some people need medication for mental health; other individuals rarely need medication of any kind. Taking proper care of your mind-body connection is a new level of responsibility that can give you a better sense of purpose and greater confidence. You have the opportunity to educate yourself on your own mental and physical needs. Make sure you allow yourself time to restore your health; it is a process. In sobriety, not only are you changing your behaviors, your thought processes, and your beliefs, but your medical health is also changing. Do not give up! Give yourself time and embrace these changes. Things will get challenging and stressful, so take your focus and energy and apply them to your new, healthier lifestyle.

QUESTIONS

1. When you have a negative mind-set, what type of physical problems occur?

____

____

____

2. What information are you providing to your doctors or medical personnel? Reflect on the questions from the book. Make sure you are being honest with yourself.

3. When you allow yourself to not forgive yourself or others, you have higher health risks. What do you need to forgive yourself and/or others for? Be specific.

4. What are your own thoughts and beliefs when it comes to over-the-counter drugs?

5. Are you experiencing any pain? What are you doing about it? What concerns do you have about how pain (both physical and emotional) could affect your sobriety?

6. What are some healthy habits you have in your life today, and what are some you need to add?

CHAPTER TEN

Aftercare Options

Researching and entering treatment can be challenging enough, but you aren't finished yet! In fact, you will always be working on your sobriety, and that is why understanding aftercare is important. Aftercare is the next step you should take after treatment, and it will look different for everyone. That is what makes it complicated.

This chapter uses a good example to demonstrate how quickly you can lose something you have worked hard for. The story depicts a woman who went through a six-month program but ended up overdosing due to using poor judgment, wanting to please others, and being overly confident. All three of those behaviors can be dangerous. The thing to understand is that you have a choice. No one else can make you do anything. It is okay to get help, advice, and suggestions from others, but at the end of the day, you have to do what is best for you. You have a lot of options for aftercare, and each is a little different. You'll find a variety of services, such as intensive outpatient (IOP), outpatient, or sober living with support groups. In Ohio, IOP would be attending nine hours and one minute of group therapy weekly, which is normally broken up over three days (roughly three hours each day). Outpatient services range from nine hours or fewer. IOP is highly recommended because of the continued structure it can provide.

To find the right aftercare path, it can be helpful to be evaluated based on standard criteria according to the American Society of Addiction Medicine (ASAM), which assesses an individual's emotional needs, withdrawal risk, medical conditions, readiness to change, relapse prevention, and recovery environment.

As was noted earlier, aftercare plans are individualized. Someone might need to continue weekly groups to help hold him or her accountable, while someone else wants more one-on-one counseling. One-on-one counseling allows you to talk about what you are going through without a peer's feedback or response. Others appreciate peer feedback and do well with attending support meetings, such as Alcoholics Anonymous, Narcotics Anonymous, Smart Recovery, Celebrate Recovery, etc. Support meetings have been around for years and have shown success. Sober living, meanwhile, helps create a safe environment and can be paired with other aftercare options. Sober living is not an option for everyone because of other obligations at home, but again: Make sure you are doing what is best for your long-term sobriety. Returning home can be overwhelming, and if you are not prepared, you could head toward a relapse. Making a pro-and-con list to break down your options can help make your decision a little clearer.

QUESTIONS

1. Do some research in your local area to assess what aftercare options are available to you. Make a list of what the programs offer (for example: group counseling, individual counseling, sober living, support meetings, etc.).

2. What are you looking for in an aftercare program? What do you want/need?

3. Make a pro-and-con list based off your findings.

PROS	CONS

Resources

WEBSITES

SAMHSA.gov – The Substance Abuse and Mental Health Services Administration has educational materials on addiction and mental health.

CDC.gov – The Centers for Disease Control and Prevention website offers statistics and other helpful medical information about alcohol and drug abuse.

DrugAbuse.gov – The National Institute on Drug Abuse provides research-based facts and information about addiction.

NAMI.org – The National Alliance on Mental Illness website includes information and resources for seeking help and support.

AA.org – The Alcoholics Anonymous website provides information about AA and how to find meetings in your area.

NA.org – The Narcotics Anonymous website provides information about NA and how to find meetings in your area.

Al-anon.alateen.org – Al-Anon provides support for family members and loved ones of problem drinkers.

Nar-anon.org – Nar-Anon provides support for family members and loved ones of those struggling with addiction.

SmartRecovery.org – The website provides information about SMART Recovery and how to find meetings in your area.

CelebrateRecovery.com – The website provides information about Celebrate Recovery, which is a Christ-centered program, and how to find meetings in your area.

BOOKS AND ARTICLES

American Psychiatric Association. *Diagnostic and Statistical Manual of Mental Disorders (5th Edition).* Washington, D.C.: American Psychiatric Publishing, 2013.

Blanco, C., Okuda, M., Wang, S., Liu, S., and Olfson, M. (2014). "Testing the Drug Substitution Switching-Addictions Hypothesis." *JAMA Psychiatry*, 71(11), 1246. doi:10.1001/jamapsychiatry.2014.1206

Foote, Jeffrey, Carrie Wilkens, Nicole Kosanke, and Stephanie Higgs. *Beyond Addiction: How Science and Kindness Help People Change.* New York: Scribner, 2014.

Frankl, Viktor. *Man's Search for Meaning.* Boston: Beacon Press, 2006.

Glasner-Edwards, Suzette. *The Addiction Recovery Skills Workbook: Changing Addictive Behaviors Using CBT, Mindfulness, and Motivational Interviewing Techniques*. Oakland, Calif.: New Harbinger Publications, 2016.

James, John W. and Russell, Friedman. *The Grief Recovery Handbook: 20th Anniversary Edition*. N.p.: HarperCollins, 2009.

Johns Hopkins Medicine. "Forgiveness: Your Health Depends on It," HopkinsMedicine.org, accessed February 6, 2018.

Kübler-Ross, Elisabeth. *On Death and Dying: What the Dying Have to Teach Doctors, Nurses, Clergy and Their Own Families*. London: Routledge, 2009.

Mayer, Emran. *The Mind-Gut Connection: How the Hidden Conversation within Our Bodies Impacts Our Mood, Our Choices, and Our Overall Health*. New York: Harper Wave, 2016.

Sheff, David. *Beautiful Boy: A Father's Journey Through His Son's Addiction*. New York: Mariner, 2008.

Spiegelman, Erica. *Rewired: A Bold New Approach to Addiction and Recovery*. Hobart, New York: Hatherleigh Press, 2015.

Williams, Rebecca E., and Julie S. Kraft. *The Mindfulness Workbook for Addiction: A Guide to Coping with the Grief, Stress, and Anger that Trigger Addictive Behaviors*. Oakland, Calif.: New Harbinger Publications, 2012.

ADDITIONAL BOOKS BY KICAM PROJECTS

Adams Recovery Center. *Accept, Reflect, Commit: Your First Steps to Addiction Recovery*. Georgetown, Ohio: KiCam Projects, 2017.

Adams Recovery Center. *Addiction, Recovery, Change: A How-To Manual for Successfully Navigating Sobriety*. Georgetown, Ohio: KiCam Projects, 2016.

Adams Recovery Center. *Assess, Rebuild, Connect: Creating a New Life Beyond Addiction*. Georgetown, Ohio: KiCam Projects, 2018.

Leder, Sharon. *The Fix: A Father's Secrets, A Daughter's Search*. Georgetown, Ohio: KiCam Projects, 2017.

Thorngren, John T. *Salvation on Death Row: The Pamela Perillo Story*. Georgetown, Ohio: KiCam Projects, 2018.

PAGES FOR JOURNALING